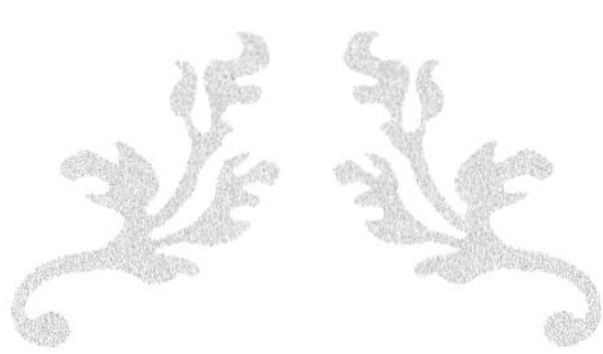

The Mind-Body Connection

Nutrition's Role in Cognitive Health

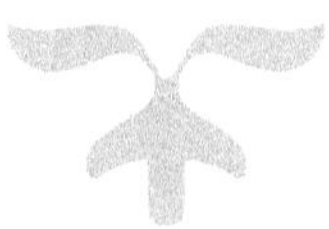

Eliza Morgan

The complicated interaction between a person's mental and physical states—known as the mind-body connection—highlights the influence of psychological processes on physical health. Over time, this idea has changed and influenced conversations about integrative therapies, holistic health, and psychosomatic medicine. In addition to treating physical illnesses, therapeutic techniques like mindfulness meditation, yoga, and cognitive behavioral therapy work to improve mental health. Nonetheless, the medical community's historical division of mind and body has resulted in an undervaluation of the importance of mental health, and methodological problems in research have increased suspicion. awareness mental and physical health still requires an awareness of the mind-body link.

Contents

INTRODUCTION

A. Overview of the Mind-Body Connection

The intricate interaction between mental and emotional states and physical health is known as the "mind-body connection," which emphasizes how attitudes, feelings, and thoughts can affect physiological well-being and vice versa. Numerous academic fields, including as psychology, neuroscience, and psychoneuroimmunology, have examined this idea, proving its applicability in comprehending health and illness in both historical and modern contexts. The interconnection of the neurological, endocrine, and immunological systems has been demonstrated by research in psychoneuroimmunology, indicating that emotional and mental states can have a significant influence on immune function. Good feelings are linked to stronger immune responses, whereas long-term stress and bad feelings can cause a number of health problems, including high blood pressure and compromised immunity to disease.

The degree to which mental states affect physical health is still up for debate, despite its long-standing acceptance. Physical symptoms like chronic pain and weariness as well as emotional problems like worry and mood swings can result from imbalances in the mind-body connection. Effective strategies to use the mind-body link for improved health, reducing symptoms of stress, anxiety, and depression, and encouraging a more balanced state of being include mindfulness, meditation, and cognitive-behavioral therapy. Participating in these activities on a regular basis can enhance emotional control and potentially alter brain morphology.

B. Importance of Nutrition in Brain Health

A vital component of total neurological well-being, brain health affects mood and cognitive performance. To maximize brain function and stave off cognitive decline, a diet rich in vital nutrients—like vitamins, antioxidants, and omega-3 fatty acids—must be well-balanced. Fatty fish, almonds, berries, and whole grains are important meals that improve cognitive function because they include essential nutrients that improve memory and focus. The quality of sleep, physical activity, and stress reduction are examples of lifestyle variables that have a big impact on cognitive results. Frequent exercise increases blood flow to the brain and triggers the production of chemicals that protect it from injury, while getting enough sleep is necessary for toxin removal and memory consolidation. Stress management is a known factor in cognitive impairment and neurodegenerative illnesses. Mindfulness techniques can assist reduce stress.

Despite the growing recognition of the importance of nutrition in brain health, challenges remain in public awareness and dietary adherence. Understanding the complexity of nutritional influences on brain health can help mitigate risks associated with cognitive decline, making it a critical area of study in both health and nutrition fields.

The goal of this book is to take a deep dive into the fascinating world of cognitive nutrition, carefully examining the impact of certain foods and eating patterns on brain function and emotional well-being. By understanding the important connection between food and mental performance, readers will learn how to use the power of food to improve memory, focus, and overall mental health. Ultimately, this book is designed to help people make food choices that not only support their physical health but also promote mental health and emotional balance.

CHAPTER 1.

The Science Behind the Mind-Body Connection

A.Understanding the Gut-Brain Axis

The digestive system—also referred to as the "second brain"—and the central nervous system are connected by the gut-brain axis, a two-way communication network that is critical to preserving mental and cognitive health. The large ecology of bacteria, viruses, and fungus that live in the gut, known as the gut microbiome, has an impact on this intricate system. These microbes are crucial for digesting, but they also regulate the synthesis of neurotransmitters, alter immunological responses, and maintain the integrity of the brain.

The vague nerve, immune system signals, and hormone signals are some of the channels via which the gut and brain can connect. The synthesis of neurotransmitters is among the most significant methods. For example, over 90% of the body's serotonin, a neurotransmitter connected to the regulation of breathing and well-being, happens in the gut. The number of beneficial bacteria in the gut microbiome directly affects mood-regulating substances like dopamine and gamma-aminobutyric acid (GABA), which in turn control emotions like stress, anxiety, and intelligence.

The gut's ability to communicate with the brain is compromised when gut health declines, which is typically brought on by poor diet, antibiotic usage, or consistent stress. This can result in diseases like "leaky gut," in which the gut lining swells and permits toxins and inflammatory substances to enter the circulation, ultimately altering brain function. Studies reveal a connection between mental health issues like anxiety, depression, and even cognitive decline with an imbalance in the gut flora. Eating foods high in fiber, probiotics (found in foods yeasts like yogurt and kimchi), and prebiotics (found in foods like onions, garlic, and bananas) can help improve gut health by bringing the gut flora back into equilibrium. Better cognitive performance and emotional well-being are supported by this strengthening of the gut-brain axis.

This can result in diseases like "leaky gut," in which the gut lining swells and permits toxins and inflammatory substances to enter the circulation, ultimately altering brain function. Studies reveal a connection between mental health issues like anxiety, depression, and even cognitive decline with an imbalance in the gut flora. Eating foods high in fiber, probiotics (found in foods yeasts like yogurt and kimchi), and prebiotics (found in foods like onions, garlic, and bananas) can help improve gut health by bringing the gut flora back into equilibrium. Better cognitive performance and emotional well-being are supported by this strengthening of the gut-brain axis.

B.Neurotransmitters and Diet

Chemical messengers called neurotransmitters are essential for controlling behavior, emotion, and perception. Maintaining appropriate levels of the most well-known neurotransmitters—serotonin, dopamine, and GABA—is critical for mental clarity, mood stability, and general cognitive function. These neurotransmitters are highly influenced by the nutrition we eat. The "happiness hormone," serotonin, is intimately related to emotions of balance and well-being. Depression, anxiety, and sleep difficulties are linked to low serotonin levels. The body naturally produces serotonin, but some foods, particularly those high in tryptophan (an amino acid that acts as a precursor to serotonin), aid in this process.

Tryptophan is found in foods including turkey, eggs, nuts, and seeds. Tryptophan raises serotonin levels in the brain when it combines with carbs. Another significant neurotransmitter that is essential for motivation, reward, and focus is dopamine. Low dopamine levels have been associated with symptoms like sadness, ADHD, and motivation issues. Tyrosine is one of the nutrients needed to produce dopamine, and it can be found in foods like fish, poultry, and dairy. Fruits and vegetables, which are high in antioxidants, shield the brain from oxidative stress, which can harm dopamine-producing neurons. The relaxing neurotransmitter GABA has a crucial role in lowering anxiety and encouraging relaxation.

Foods high in magnesium, like leafy greens, nuts, and seeds, boost the production of GABA and support emotional equilibrium. In a similar vein, probiotics found in fermented foods like kimchi and yogurt encourage the creation of GABA in the stomach, which supports mental health even more. A person's mood, focus, and ability to prevent cognitive deterioration can all be enhanced by following dietary patterns that support the creation and control of these neurotransmitters. Conversely, diets heavy in processed foods and dietary deficits might result in neurotransmitter abnormalities and psychological issues.

C. Inflammation and Cognitive Decline

Chronic inflammation is becoming more widely acknowledged as a major risk factor for neurological illnesses like Alzheimer's and a major contributor to issues with both physical and mental health. As the immune system of the body reacts to damaging stimuli like infections or injuries, inflammation results. Acute inflammation is a natural component of the healing process, but chronic inflammation can harm tissues, cells, and even the functioning of the brain over an extended period of time. Chronic inflammation can be brought on by poor eating habits, such as consuming a lot of processed foods, refined carbohydrates, and unhealthy fats. These meals frequently result in an excess of pro-inflammatory chemicals, like cytokines, which can impair cognitive performance by crossing the blood-brain barrier.

This can eventually result in oxidative stress and the development of toxic plaques in the brain, which are linked to dementias like Alzheimer's. It has been demonstrated that omega-3 fatty acids, which are present in foods like walnuts, flaxseeds, and fatty fish (like salmon and sardines), reduce inflammation and stop cognitive deterioration. These fats boost neuroplasticity, which is the brain's capacity to adapt and create new connections even as we age, and have anti-inflammatory qualities. They also preserve the integrity of brain cells. Antioxidants, which are present in dark chocolate, green tea, and berries, can help combat inflammation by scavenging free radicals, which are unstable chemicals that cause cellular damage and accelerate aging and cognitive decline.

Chronic inflammation can be avoided by eating a diet high in whole foods and nutrients that reduce inflammation, promoting both mental and physical well-being. An anti-inflammatory diet and a reduction in processed food consumption may shield your brain from the long-term effects of inflammation, hence lowering your risk of memory loss, cognitive decline, and neurodegenerative illnesses.

Knowing the science behind inflammation, neurotransmitters, and the gut-brain axis reveals the significant influence of nutrition on cognitive function. People can greatly enhance their long-term brain health, mental clarity, and mood by adopting mindful dietary choices.

CHAPTER 2.

Nutrients Essential for Cognitive Health

A.Omega-3 Fatty Acids

Omega-3 fatty acids are one of the most important nutrients for brain health, playing a key role in the structure and function of brain cells. These fats, especially docosahexaenoic acid (DHA) and eicosatetraenoic acid (EPA), are key components of brain cell membranes, ensuring fluidity and optimal communication between neurons. Adequate amounts of DHA and EPA are important for neuroplasticity, which supports the brain's ability to adapt and form new connections, a key component of learning, memory, and overall cognitive resilience.

Omega-3 fatty acids also have anti-inflammatory properties, protecting the brain from inflammation-related damage and cognitive decline. Research has shown that a diet rich in omega-3 fatty acids can reduce the risk of neurodegenerative diseases such as Alzheimer's, improve mood by supporting neurotransmitter function, and even relieve symptoms of depression.

<u>***Sources and Recommendations***</u>

The best sources of omega-3 fatty acids are fatty fish such as salmon, mackerel, sardines, and anchovies. Plant sources such as flaxseeds, chia seeds, and walnuts contain alpha-linolenic acid (ALA), a precursor to DHA and EPA, although it is less converted by the body. For optimal brain health, adults are recommended to consume at least two servings of fatty fish per week, with approximately 250-500 mg of EPA and DHA combined per day.

For those who do not eat fish, high-quality fish oil or algae supplements are effective alternatives to ensure adequate omega-3 intake.

B.Antioxidants and Brain Protection

Antioxidants are substances that assist in shielding the brain against oxidative stress, which arises from an imbalance between the body's capacity to eliminate free radicals—unstable molecules that have the potential to cause cell damage—and the radicals themselves. Oxidative stress is a factor in aging, cognitive loss, and the onset of neurodegenerative diseases such as Alzheimer's disease over time.

Flavonoids and vitamins C and E are among the most potent antioxidants that can shield brain tissue. In addition to being essential for the production of neurotransmitters like dopamine and serotonin, vitamin C is also necessary for combating free radicals in the brain. It is well known that vitamin E, especially when present in its unprocessed form as alpha-tocopherol, shields cell membranes from oxidative damage.

Due to their extreme sensitivity to oxidative stress, neurons require specific attention to ensure their health.

Moreover, the plant-based antioxidants known as flavonoids, which are present in a variety of vibrant fruits and vegetables, have neuroprotective advantages. These substances improve blood flow to the brain, lower inflammation, and foster neuroplasticity, all of which improve memory and learning.

Antioxidant-Rich Diets

i.   Antioxidant-rich foods include:
ii. Vitamin C can be found in bell peppers, citrus fruits, berries, and leafy greens.
iii. Vitamin E is found in avocado, almonds, seeds, and spinach.
iv. Flavonoids include citrus fruits, dark chocolate, berries (strawberries, blueberries), and tea (black and green).
v.   Including a range of these foods high in antioxidants in the diet can help prevent age-related brain damage and support cognitive lifespan.

C.B-Vitamins and Mental Clarity

B-vitamins are necessary to sustain energy levels, emotional management, and cognitive performance. These vitamins—B6, B9 (folate), and B12 in particular—are essential for the healthy creation of neurotransmitters and the upkeep of nerve cells in the brain.

The three chemicals that control mood, stress, and cognitive focus—serotonin, dopamine, and GABA—are produced in part by vitamin B6. Sufficient intake of B6 can help avoid mood fluctuations and mental exhaustion.

Folate, or vitamin B9, is essential for brain growth and cognitive function because it promotes DNA synthesis and cell repair. Additionally, homocysteine, an amino acid that raises the risk of dementia and cognitive decline at high levels, is metabolized by folate.

The myelin sheath, the covering that protects nerve cells, depends on vitamin B12 to remain healthy. It is also required for the synthesis of red blood cells, which guarantees that the brain gets enough oxygen to function at its best.

Deficits in certain B-complex vitamins have been associated with depression, memory problems, and mental fog. As a result, keeping levels appropriate is essential for emotional equilibrium and mental clarity.

Top Dietary B-Vitamin Sources

i.   Fish, poultry, potatoes, bananas, and fortified cereals are good sources of vitamin B6.

ii.   Vegetables high in folate include beans, peas, and fortified grains.

iii.   Meat, fish, eggs, and dairy products are examples of animal items high in vitamin B12. For vegetarians and vegans, fortified plant-based substitutes are available.

D.Minerals and Trace Elements

Zinc, magnesium, and iron are examples of minerals and trace elements that have a major impact on cognitive function, influencing anything from mood management to memory and focus.

The function of neurotransmitters and the control of neuronal communication are both impacted by zinc. Deficits in zinc have been related to depression and ADHD as well as poor cognitive development. Additionally, neurogenesis—the process of creating new neurons—is supported by zinc and is crucial for memory and learning.

Magnesium is necessary for brain cell energy generation and nerve transmission. Additionally, it aids in nervous system regulation, which lowers anxiety and encourages relaxation. Fatigue, emotional issues, and cognitive impairment are linked to magnesium shortage.

Iron deficiency can cause anemia, exhaustion, and impaired cognitive function, particularly in women.

For the best possible physical and mental health, it is imperative to consume a diet balanced in these minerals. Any one of these minerals taken in excess or insufficiently might cause imbalances that impair cognitive function and mental clarity.

Where to Find Vital Minerals

i. Beans, meat, oysters, and pumpkin seeds are good sources of zinc.
ii. Grains, cashews, almonds, and leafy greens are good sources of magnesium.
iii. Iron-rich foods include lentils, red meat, spinach, and fortified cereals.

Maintaining a diet high in these minerals can enhance mental health generally, prevent mental tiredness, and enhance cognitive function.

These vital nutrients—antioxidants, B-vitamins, crucial minerals, and omega-3 fatty acids—can greatly increase mental clarity, prevent cognitive decline, and maintain brain health when included in a regular diet. People can support cognitive longevity and sustain good mental function throughout their lives by choosing well-informed dietary choice

CHAPTER 3.

Dietary Patterns and Mental Health

A.The Mediterranean Diet

The many health benefits of the Mediterranean diet are well known, especially in terms of enhancing cognitive function and lowering the risk of mental decline. This diet is low in processed foods, sweets, and red meat and high on whole foods including fruits, vegetables, whole grains, legumes, nuts, seeds, and lean proteins like fish. Its focus on whole, nutrient-dense foods makes it an effective tool for preserving mental clarity and lowering the risk of neurodegenerative illnesses.

The Mediterranean diet promotes mental wellness in a number of ways. First off, its high omega-3 fatty acid content from fish and olive oil enhances neurotransmitter activity, lowers inflammation, and preserves the structural integrity of brain cells—all vital for cognitive function.

Furthermore, a diet high in fruits and vegetables provides antioxidants that shield brain cells from oxidative stress and shield neurons from harm. Additionally, by fostering neuroplasticity the brain's capacity to adjust, create new connections, and heal from injury these antioxidants aid with memory and learning.

Studies have repeatedly demonstrated that those following a Mediterranean diet are less likely to experience cognitive decline, dementia, or Alzheimer's disease. According to studies, this diet not only improves executive function and memory, but it also reduces the risk of anxiety and sadness. A body that supports both physical and mental well-being is fostered by the Mediterranean diet's balanced consumption of fiber, healthy fats, and vitamins.

Important Diets and Activities for Optimal Brain Function

i. Omega-3-rich foods include walnuts, olive oil, and fatty fish (salmon, mackerel, and sardines).
ii. Foods high in antioxidants include citrus fruits, almonds, tomatoes, berries, and leafy greens.
iii. Legumes and whole grains, such as quinoa, barley, lentils, and chickpeas
iv. Fish, poultry, beans, and lentils are examples of lean proteins.
v. Good fats: avocados, nuts, seeds, and olive oil

By incorporating these essential nutrients and adhering to the Mediterranean diet's principles, one can considerably improve brain function and foster long-term mental clarity.

B.Plant-Based Diets and Brain Performance

Plant-based diets have been linked to several health advantages, such as enhanced mental and emotional well-being. These diets emphasize entire foods produced from plants while reducing or eliminating animal products. In order to enhance cognitive function, the plant-based diet places a strong emphasis on consuming fruits, vegetables, whole grains, legumes, nuts, and seeds—all of which are high in fiber, vitamins, and minerals.

Reducing inflammation and oxidative stress, two factors that lead to cognitive decline, is one of the main advantages of plant-based diets. Antioxidants, which shield neurons from harm and support normal brain aging, are abundant in plant-based diets. These include flavonoids, polyphenols, and vitamins C and E.

Additionally, these diets typically contain more unsaturated fats from foods like avocados, almonds, and seeds, which are good for the health of the brain, and less saturated fats, which are linked to an increased risk of cognitive impairment.

A diet high in plant-based fiber also helps to maintain gut health by feeding good gut flora. Because of the gut-brain axis, mental health is intimately associated with a healthy gut flora. According to studies, people who follow plant-based diets typically experience reduced rates of anxiety, sadness, and cognitive decline. This is probably because these diets have a good effect on both the stomach and the brain.

Studies Backing Plant-Based Diets for Mental Sharpness The benefits of plant-based diets for cognitive function have been shown in numerous research.

Studies Backing Plant-Based Diets for Mental Sharpness
The benefits of plant-based diets for cognitive function have been shown in numerous research. For instance, studies have shown that those who eat vegetarian or veganism frequently do better cognitively, especially in areas like memory and attention. According to a 2019 study that was published in the Journal of the American Medical Association, people who ate a plant-based diet were less likely to age with dementia and cognitive impairment.

Important Components of a Plant-Based Diet for Brain Health

i. Berries, citrus fruits, and dark green vegetables are great sources of antioxidants.
ii. Whole grains: barley, brown rice, quinoa, and oats
iii. Nuts, seeds, avocados, and olive oil are good sources of fat.
iv. Beans and legumes: black beans, chickpeas, and lentils
v. Plant-based proteins: beans, edamame, tempeh, and tofu
vi. People can preserve their brain from age-related degeneration, improve their mood, and increase cognitive clarity by concentrating on full, unprocessed plant foods.

C.The Effects of Processed Foods on the Brain

The current diet can be harmful to brain function since it frequently contains high levels of processed foods, refined sugars, unhealthy fats, and artificial additives. Usually lacking in vital nutrients, these foods are rich in compounds that exacerbate inflammation and oxidative stress, impairing cognitive function and raising the risk of mental health issues.

Sugar and Cognitive Processes

Consuming too much sugar, especially in the form of sweetened beverages, candies, and baked goods, can have a detrimental effect on one's cognitive health. Sugar causes insulin levels to surge, which over time can result in insulin resistance also known as "type 3 diabetes" a condition that is associated with a higher risk of Alzheimer's disease and brain damage.

Bad Fats and Cognitive Regression

Diets heavy in trans and saturated fats, which are frequently found in fried foods, processed snacks, and fast food, can harm neurons' structural integrity and cause inflammation, which can affect brain function. According to research, those who eat a diet heavy in unhealthy fats are more prone to develop dementia and other neurodegenerative disorders, as well as to experience cognitive loss.

Artificial Sweeteners and Emotional Well-Being

Artificial additives included in many processed meals, like colorants, flavor enhancers, and preservatives, can be detrimental to the health of the brain. For instance, some artificial sweeteners have been connected to mood and anxiety disorders, while colorants and preservatives may be a factor in hyperactivity and concentration issues, especially in young children.

Negative Dietary Decisions' Long-Term Effects on Mental Health Poor eating habits that involve consuming processed meals often over time might cause long-term harm to the health of the brain. Processed food consumption can raise one's risk of mental health conditions such anxiety, depression, and cognitive loss. Research has indicated that those who follow a Western diet, which is high in processed foods, sugar, and unhealthy fats, are less likely to perform cognitively and are more likely to suffer from mental health problems than persons who eat a diet rich in whole foods and nutrients.

People can safeguard their brain health, increase mental clarity, and lower their chance of developing long-term cognitive impairments by avoiding processed foods and putting an emphasis on full, nutrient-rich foods.

For mental and cognitive health, adopting plant-based and Mediterranean diets, as well as staying away from processed foods, can have significant advantages. We may dramatically improve brain function, emotional health, and long-term cognitive resilience by choosing our foods carefully.

CHAPTER 4.

Nutrition for Mental Disorders

A.Diet and Depression

An intricate mental health disorder, depression is impacted by a range of elements, such as lifestyle, environment, and heredity. Recent studies have demonstrated a robust association between depression risk and food quality, emphasizing the part that nutrition plays in the development and treatment of this mental illness. Unhealthy eating patterns, especially those heavy in sugar, processed foods, and bad fats, are linked to an increased risk of depression. Conversely, diets high in whole, nutrient-dense foods can help lower the chance of developing depression and lessen its symptoms.

The Connection Between Depression Risk and Diet Quality

An elevated intake of refined carbohydrates, sugar, and trans fats can stimulate oxidative stress and inflammation, two factors associated with the onset of depression. Depression is frequently accompanied by higher levels of inflammatory markers, such as C-reactive protein (CRP), which suggests that inflammation brought on by poor diet may contribute to the condition.

Furthermore, dietary deficiencies, such as low levels of magnesium, B vitamins, and omega-3 fatty acids, can worsen depressive symptoms by upsetting neurotransmitter balance and causing more oxidative damage to brain tissue.

On the other hand, whole food-focused diets, like the Mediterranean diet, are linked to decreased rates of depression. A lot of fruits, vegetables, whole grains, legumes, lean proteins (like fish), healthy fats (like olive oil), and whole grains are all part of this diet. These meals offer vital nutrients that promote neurotransmitter activity and brain health, lowering inflammation and promoting mood stability.

Dietary Techniques for Depression Management and Prevention

Omega-3 Fatty Acids: These fats, which are present in walnuts, flaxseeds, and fatty fish, support the construction and function of the brain and are involved in the control of serotonin. It has been demonstrated that taking omega-3 supplements, especially EPA, can lessen the symptoms of depression. B-Vitamins: B12 and folate (B9) are essential for mood modulation and brain function. Depression and low levels of certain vitamins are related. Foods that assist guarantee proper intake include beans, leafy greens, fortified cereals, and animal products. Antioxidants: Fruits and vegetables contain flavonoids, vitamin C, and vitamin E, which help lower oxidative stress, which is linked to depression. Eating meals high in antioxidants on a regular basis can help stabilize your mood. Whole grains, nuts, seeds, and leafy greens are among the foods high in magnesium. Probiotics: The relationship between gut health and mental health, especially depression, is becoming more widely acknowledged. Eating foods high in probiotics, such as kefir, yogurt, and fermented vegetables, can help maintain a healthy gut-brain axis, which in turn can help boost mood.

B. Anxiety and the Role of Nutrients

One of the most prevalent mental health issues is anxiety disorders, and new research suggests that food has a significant impact on both preventing and treating anxiety symptoms. A healthy diet can help control the neurotransmitters that affect stress and mood, and some nutrients are especially good at lowering anxiety.

Foods and Nutrients that Help Lower the Symptoms of Anxiety

i. Magnesium: This mineral is necessary for the hypothalamic-pituitary-adrenal (HPA) axis, which controls the body's reaction to stress, as well as for relaxing the neurological system. Having too little magnesium can make you feel more anxious. Nuts, seeds, legumes, and leafy greens are among the foods high in magnesium that can help reduce symptoms.

ii. Omega-3 Fatty Acids: By lowering inflammation and enhancing the health of neurotransmitters, these vital fats—which may be found in fatty fish, chia seeds, and flaxseeds—help regulate mood. Research indicates that those who have enough omega-3 fatty acids typically experience reduced anxiety.

iii. B-Vitamins: The synthesis of neurotransmitters like serotonin and GABA, which both aid in mood regulation, depends on vitamins B6 and B12. Stress and anxiety may be exacerbated by deficiencies in certain vitamins. Good sources include whole grains, seafood, poultry, and fortified

iv. L-theanine: This amino acid, which is present in green tea, has been demonstrated to increase alpha brain waves, which in turn help to promote relaxation and lessen anxiety. Drinking green tea on a regular basis can help you focus better and manage

v. Probiotics: Studies indicate that a balanced gut flora may improve mental health by lowering anxiety symptoms. Foods high in probiotics, such as kimchi, sauerkraut, and yogurt, can facilitate gut-brain contact and encourage a calmer mental state.

Managing Anxiety and Blood Sugar with a Healthy Diet

The control of blood sugar is one of the frequently disregarded causes of worry. Anxiety, irritability, and mood swings can be brought on by abrupt increases and decreases in blood sugar, which are frequently brought on by eating processed carbs and sugary meals. In order to keep blood sugar levels steady, you must:

Consume well-balanced meals that include complex carbohydrates, protein, and healthy fats to avoid blood sugar

Steer clear of processed sugars: Reduce your intake of sugary drinks and snacks in favor of whole fruits or nuts. Eat frequently: Missing meals can cause blood sugar levels to plummet, which can heighten agitation and anxiety. Blood sugar can be stabilized throughout the day with regular, well-balanced meals.

C. Cognitive Decline and Alzheimer's Prevention

A major issue for the aging population is dementia, including Alzheimer's disease and other types. Because specific nutrients and dietary patterns have been found to enhance brain function and delay the advancement of neurodegenerative illnesses, nutrition plays a vital role in minimizing the risk of cognitive decline.

Dietary Strategies for Lowering Alzheimer's and Dementia risk

   i. The Mediterranean Diet: It has been shown in studies to reduce the risk of cognitive impairment by thirty to forty percent. Antioxidants, anti-inflammatory substances, and healthy fats included in this diet, which is high in fruits, vegetables, seafood, whole grains, and olive oil, promote brain function and stave off the onset of dementia.

ii. The MIND diet: Referred to as the Mediterranean-DASH Diet Intervention for Neurodegenerative Delay, is a cross between the DASH and Mediterranean diets that focuses on foods that are good for the brain. It limits red meat, butter, cheese, and sweets while emphasizing leafy greens, berries, nuts, whole grains, and seafood. According to studies, the MIND diet greatly reduces the risk of Alzheimer's in participants.

iii. Ketogenic Diet: The high-fat, low-carbohydrate ketogenic diet has demonstrated potential in preliminary studies as a means of preserving brain function by supplying ketones, an alternative energy source. Though further research is required, this diet may help those with Alzheimer's disease perform better cognitively and in terms of memory.

The Function of Nutrients, Fats, and Vitamins in Sustaining Cognitive Longevity

i. DHA is a form of omega-3 fatty acid that is essential to the structural integrity of brain cells. Consuming enough omega-3 fatty acids from fish or supplements promotes cognitive performance, preserves brain structure, and lowers the risk of Alzheimer's.

ii. B-vitamin-rich foods like leafy greens, beans, and animal products can help reduce this risk.

Antioxidants: Vitamins C and E are examples of antioxidants that shield brain tissue from oxidative stress and damage from free radicals. Consuming foods high in antioxidants, such as citrus fruits, almonds, and berries, can help avert cognitive deterioration.

iii. Polyphenols: Foods high in polyphenols, such as dark chocolate, red wine, and green tea, have been demonstrated to enhance memory and shield brain tissue from aging-related deterioration.

A nutrient-dense diet high in whole foods and healthy fats can lower an individual's risk of Alzheimer's and help them retain their cognitive abilities well into old life.

Mental health and cognitive function are greatly impacted by nutrition, which can affect anything from anxiety and mood to the long-term risk of developing neurodegenerative disorders like Alzheimer's. By making thoughtful food choices, people can safeguard their mental health, avoid mental illnesses, and extend their cognitive lifespan.

CHAPTER 5.

Creating a Nutritional Plan for Cognitive Health

A.Building a Brain-Healthy Diet

Maintaining cognitive health is greatly aided by a solid nutritional base. Creating a diet that is good for the brain requires learning about the essential elements that support mental health, practicing mindful eating, and researching supplements that might improve cognitive function.

Essential Elements of a Mind-Body Balanced Diet

i. Good Fats: Fish (salmon, sardines), flaxseeds, and walnuts are good sources of omega-3 fatty acids, which are essential for brain health. They lessen inflammation and facilitate brain cell-to-brain communication.

ii. Antioxidants: Rich in antioxidants, berries, dark leafy greens, and other fruits and vegetables shield the brain from oxidative stress, which over time can cause cognitive impairment. Whole Grains: The main energy source for the brain, glucose, is released steadily by foods like quinoa, brown rice, and oats, supporting mental clarity and vigor.

iii. Lean Proteins: Foods high in protein, such as chicken, eggs, tofu, and lentils, provide the amino acids needed to produce neurotransmitters, which elevate mood and enhance cognitive performance.

iv. Hydration: Water is essential for the health of the brain.

v. Techniques for Meal Planning with Cognitive Support

vi. Balanced Meals: To maintain energy levels and cognitive performance throughout the day, include a variety of complex carbohydrates, lean proteins, and healthy fats in each meal.

vii. Colorful Plate: To guarantee a range of vitamins and antioxidants that support brain health, try to have a diversity of colors on your plate from fruits and vegetables.

viii. Snacks for Brain Power: Steer clear of sugar-filled goodies and opt instead for snacks that contain a combination of healthy fats and antioxidants, such as nuts, seeds, or a piece of dark chocolate.

ix. Consistency: Eating regular meals at regular intervals throughout the day keeps your brain nourished, which enhances focus and mental clarity. It also prevents energy dips.

B. Mindful Eating for Mental Clarity

How Eating With Mindfulness Improves Cognitive Function

i. Being present during meals and focusing on the tastes, textures, and sensations of the food, along with your body's signals of hunger and fullness, are all part of mindful eating.

ii. According to studies, practicing mindfulness can enhance one's capacity for memory, concentration, and decision-making. Being mindful of what and how you eat can help you avoid overindulging, which frequently results in fatigue and diminished mental clarity.

Including Mindful Activities in Everyday Meals

i. Eat Slowly: Give your food enough time to be completely chewed and enjoyed. This helps with digestion and allows your brain enough time to register fullness.

ii. Eliminate All Distractions: Steer clear of multitasking when eating, such as watching TV or using your phone. Rather, give your meal your whole attention, as this will help your brain recognize the food's nutritious content.

iii. Thank You for the Food: Take a time to appreciate the food that is in front of you before you begin each meal. By refocusing your attention on the act of feeding your body, this technique might help you develop a stronger bond with the eating process.

iv. Recognize Cues of Hunger and Fullness: Keep a watchful eye out for bodily cues indicating hunger and fullness. This can help you avoid overeating by teaching your brain to detect appropriate portion sizes over time.

C. Supplements for Brain Health

An Overview of Cognitive Supplements Based on Evidence

i. DHA and EPA,: These often known as omega-3 fatty acids, are known to play a part in brain formation and maintenance. They also promote cognitive function and may lower the risk of neurodegenerative illnesses.

ii. Vitamin B: These vitamins, especially folic acid, B6, and B12, are essential for brain health and may help prevent cognitive aging and memory loss.
Vitamin D: Supplementing with vitamin D can be helpful, particularly for communities with little sun exposure, as low levels of the vitamin have been related to cognitive impairment.

iii. Antioxidants, such as vitamins C and E: Antioxidants have been shown in certain studies to enhance memory and decrease the aging process of the brain by shielding brain cells from oxidative damage.

iv.   Nootropics: Although more research is required to validate their usefulness, supplements like Ginkgo Biloba, Rhodiola Rosea, and Bacopa Monnier are frequently marketed for their ability to improve brain clarity and minimize mental tiredness.

When to Think About Supplements and How to Pick the correctives

When to Supplement: Supplementation might be a useful addition if dietary sources of important brain nutrients are insufficient. When deficits exist, such as poor omega-3 consumption in vegetarian diets or low vitamin D in areas with little sunlight, it is very helpful.

i.   Selecting Appropriate Supplements: Seek for supplements with supporting data that have undergone independent testing to ensure their potency and purity. Before beginning any new supplement regimen, always get medical advice, especially if you are taking medication or have underlying medical conditions.

ii.   Timing and Dosage: Pay attention to suggested dosages and the best times to take supplements. Certain vitamins, such as fat-soluble vitamins D and E, are better absorbed when consumed with fat-containing foods, while others may need to be taken at particular times to have the best effects.

CONCLUSION

A. Recap of the Mind-Body Connection

Maintaining cognitive health requires eating mindfully and consuming healthy fats. Mental health and brain function are supported by a well-balanced diet full of vital nutrients, such as antioxidants, whole grains, lean proteins, healthy fats, and adequate hydration. Additionally, supplements can improve brain function and fill in nutritional shortages.

B. The Future of Cognitive Nutrition

An emerging field that examines the connection between nutrition and mental health is nutritional psychiatry. Targeted nutrition may help prevent or treat mental health conditions including depression and cognitive loss, according to research. Probiotics, prebiotics, and customized nutrition may be included in future dietary recommendations to enhance brain function. Nootropic pills and functional meals are also becoming more and more popular.

C. Final Thoughts: Taking Control of Your Cognitive Health Through Diet and Lifestyle

You can walk down the path to improved cognitive wellness. Knowing how diet impacts the brain will help you make decisions that promote mental clarity, focus, and general wellbeing. You may take charge of your cognitive health by combining a nutrient-dense diet with evidence-based supplementation and mindful eating techniques. Moreover, keeping up with new developments in nutritional psychiatry can assist you in modifying your diet to reflect the most recent findings in science, guaranteeing your long-term mental and physical health.